ECZEMA DIET COOKBOOK

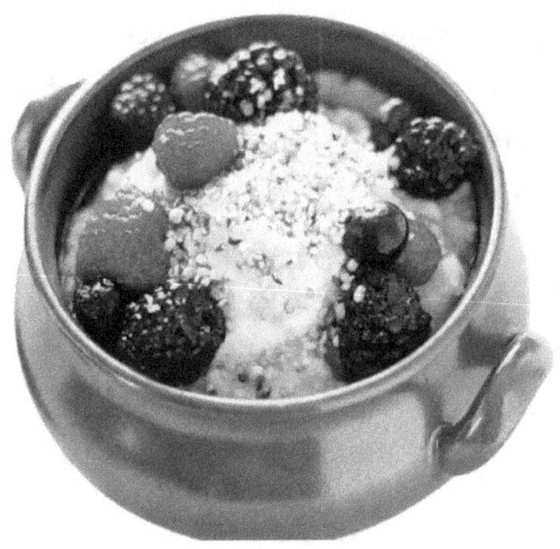

Gluten-Free Recipes to Fight Flare Ups & Itches

ALLIE NAGEL

Copyright © 2024 by Allie Nagel

DISCLAIMER

This cookbook is intended to provide general information and recipes.

The recipes provided in this cookbook are not intended to replace or be a substitute for medical advice from a physician.

The reader should consult a healthcare professional for any specific medical advice, diagnosis or treatment.

Any specific dietary advice provided in this cookbook is not intended to replace or be a substitute for medical advice from a physician.

The author is not responsible or liable for any adverse effects experienced by readers of this cookbook as a result of following the recipes or dietary advice provided.

The author makes no representations or warranties of any kind (express or implied) as to the accuracy, completeness, reliability or suitability of the recipes provided in this cookbook.

The author disclaims any and all liability for any damages arising out of the use or misuse of the recipes provided in this cookbook. The reader must also take care to ensure that the recipes provided in this cookbook are prepared and cooked safely.

The recipes provided in this cookbook are for informational purposes only and should not be used as a substitute for professional medical advice, diagnosis or treatment.

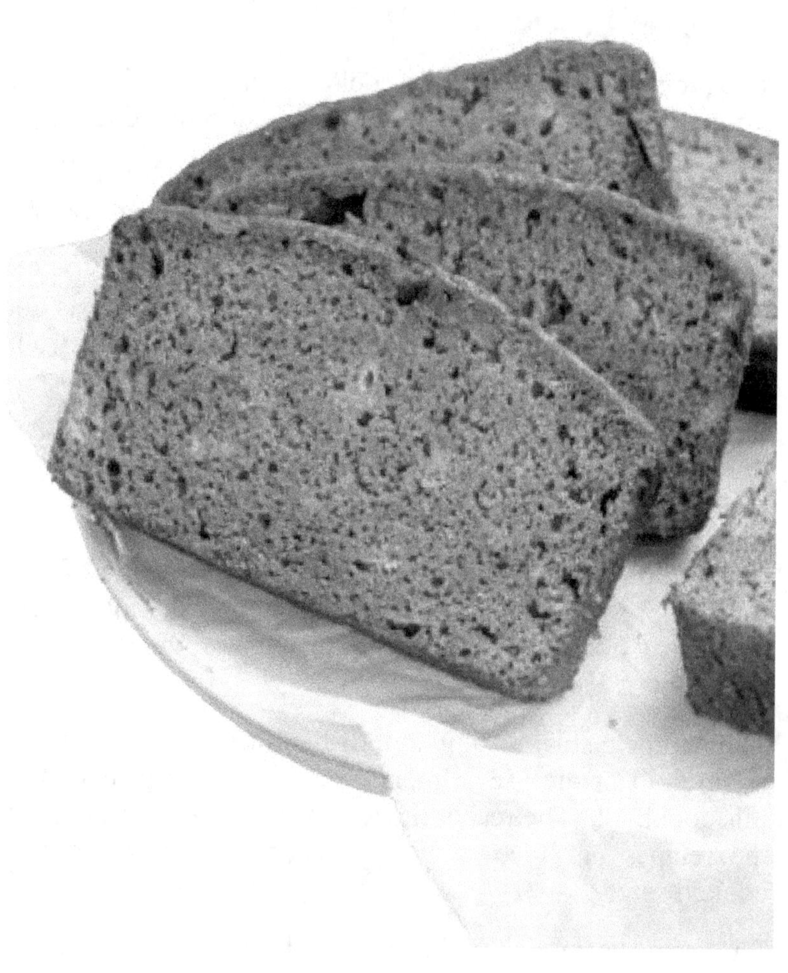

TABLE OF CONTENTS

INTRODUCTION

Eczema is a prevalent dermatological issue marked by inflammation, itchiness, and redness of the skin.

It affects people of all ages, from infants to adults, and can have a significant impact on quality of life.

Understanding the causes, symptoms, and management strategies for eczema is essential for those of you living with the condition and your caregivers.

The exact cause of eczema is not fully understood, but it is believed to involve a combination of genetic, environmental, and immune system factors.

Anyone with a family history of eczema, asthma, or allergies are at a higher risk of developing the condition. Environmental triggers such as irritants, allergens, weather changes, stress, and certain foods can exacerbate symptoms and lead to flare-ups.

Symptoms of eczema vary from person to person but often include dry, itchy skin, red or inflamed patches, rough or scaly areas, and in severe cases, oozing or crusting.

These symptoms can be uncomfortable and may interfere with daily activities and sleep, affecting both physical and emotional well-being.

Managing eczema involves a combination of preventive measures and treatment strategies aimed at relieving symptoms and preventing flare-ups.

This may include identifying and avoiding triggers, using gentle skincare products, moisturizing regularly to hydrate the skin, and practicing stress management techniques.

In some cases, topical corticosteroids, antihistamines, or immunomodulators may be prescribed by a healthcare professional to reduce inflammation and itching.

Additionally, emerging research suggests that lifestyle factors such as diet and gut health may play a role in eczema management.

Some people find relief from symptoms by following an anti-inflammatory diet rich in fruits, vegetables, omega-3 fatty acids, and probiotics, while avoiding potential triggers such as dairy, gluten, and processed foods.

CHAPTER 1

TYPES OF ECZEMA

1. **Atopic Dermatitis:** This is the most common form of eczema, often associated with a family history of allergic conditions like asthma or hay fever. It typically appears as dry, itchy patches on the skin, especially in areas such as the face, hands, elbows, and knees.

2. **Contact Dermatitis:** Contact dermatitis occurs when the skin comes into contact with an irritant or allergen, leading to inflammation and irritation. Irritant contact dermatitis is caused by exposure to substances like detergents, solvents, or chemicals, while allergic contact dermatitis results from an allergic reaction to a specific substance like latex or nickel.

3. **Seborrheic Dermatitis:** This type of eczema primarily affects the scalp, face, and upper body, causing redness, scaling, and flaking of the skin. It is commonly associated with excessive oil production

and may be exacerbated by factors such as stress, hormonal changes, or certain medications.

4. **Dyshidrotic Eczema:** Dyshidrotic eczema, also known as pompholyx, is characterized by small, fluid-filled blisters that develop on the palms of the hands, soles of the feet, or sides of the fingers. These blisters can be intensely itchy and may cause discomfort or pain.

5. **Nummular Eczema:** Nummular eczema presents as round or oval-shaped patches of inflamed, red skin that may be dry, scaly, or crusted. It often occurs on the arms, legs, or torso and may be triggered by factors such as dry skin, irritants, or stress.

6. **Stasis Dermatitis:** Stasis dermatitis typically affects the lower legs and ankles, often in individuals with poor circulation or venous insufficiency. It is characterized by swollen, itchy skin, redness, and scaling, and may lead to complications such as ulcers or infections if left untreated.

7. **Neurodermatitis:** Also known as lichen simplex chronicus, neurodermatitis is a localized form of eczema characterized by thick, leathery patches of

skin that result from repeated scratching or rubbing. It commonly occurs on the neck, wrists, ankles, or genital area and may be triggered by stress or psychological factors.

HOW THE ECZEMA DIET WORKS

The Eczema Diet, also known as the Anti-Inflammatory Diet, aims to manage eczema symptoms by reducing inflammation in the body and identifying potential dietary triggers that may exacerbate the condition. Here's how the eczema diet works:

1. **Identifying Trigger Foods:** The first step in the eczema diet is to identify potential trigger foods that may worsen eczema symptoms. Common triggers include dairy, gluten, eggs, soy, nuts, shellfish, and certain fruits and vegetables. By eliminating these foods from the diet, individuals can assess whether their eczema symptoms improve.

2. **Reducing Inflammatory Foods:** The eczema diet emphasizes reducing consumption of foods that are known to promote inflammation in the body. This includes processed foods, refined sugars, trans fats,

and excessive consumption of omega-6 fatty acids found in vegetable oils. Instead, the diet encourages whole, minimally processed foods that are rich in anti-inflammatory nutrients.

3. **Emphasizing Anti-Inflammatory Foods:** Anti-inflammatory foods play a key role in the eczema diet, as they can help reduce inflammation in the body and support overall skin health. These include fruits and vegetables, especially those high in antioxidants and phytonutrients, as well as fatty fish rich in omega-3 fatty acids, such as salmon, mackerel, and sardines.

4. **Optimizing Gut Health:** Emerging research suggests a link between gut health and eczema, with certain gastrointestinal issues contributing to the development or exacerbation of the condition. The eczema diet may include probiotic-rich foods like yogurt, kefir, and fermented vegetables to support a healthy gut microbiome.

5. **Hydration:** Adequate hydration is essential for overall skin health and may help alleviate eczema symptoms. Drinking plenty of water throughout the

day can help keep the skin hydrated and improve its ability to retain moisture.

6. **Balanced Nutrition:** The eczema diet promotes a balanced intake of nutrients, including vitamins, minerals, and essential fatty acids, to support overall health and well-being. This may involve incorporating a variety of nutrient-dense foods into the diet, such as lean proteins, whole grains, nuts, seeds, and legumes.

7. **Individualized Approach:** It's important to note that the eczema diet is not one-size-fits-all, and individual responses to specific foods can vary. Some individuals may find relief by eliminating certain trigger foods, while others may benefit from additional dietary modifications or supplementation. Consulting with a healthcare professional or registered dietitian can help individuals develop a personalized eczema diet plan tailored to their specific needs and preferences.

FOODS THAT CAN TRIGGER ECZEMA TO AVOID

1. **Dairy Products:** Cow's milk and dairy products like cheese, yogurt, and ice cream are common triggers for eczema, particularly in children. Dairy contains proteins that may trigger allergic reactions and inflammation in some individuals.

2. **Gluten-Containing Grains:** Wheat, barley, rye, and other gluten-containing grains are potential triggers for eczema, especially in individuals with gluten sensitivities or celiac disease. Gluten can contribute to inflammation and may exacerbate eczema symptoms in some people.

3. **Eggs:** Eggs are a common allergen and may trigger eczema flare-ups in susceptible individuals. Both the egg white and yolk can potentially cause allergic reactions and inflammation in some people with eczema.

4. **Soy Products:** Soybeans and soy-based products like tofu, soy milk, and soy sauce are common triggers for eczema, particularly in individuals with soy allergies. Soy contains proteins that can elicit

allergic reactions and may worsen eczema symptoms.

5. **Nuts and Seeds:** Tree nuts, such as almonds, walnuts, and cashews, as well as seeds like sesame seeds, can trigger allergic reactions and inflammation in some individuals with eczema. Peanuts, while technically legumes, can also exacerbate eczema symptoms in susceptible individuals.

6. **Shellfish:** Shellfish, including shrimp, crab, lobster, and clams, are common allergens that can trigger eczema flare-ups in sensitive individuals. Shellfish proteins can cause allergic reactions and may exacerbate inflammation in the skin.

7. **Citrus Fruits:** Citrus fruits like oranges, lemons, limes, and grapefruits contain high levels of citric acid, which can be irritating to the skin and may exacerbate eczema symptoms in some individuals.

8. **Tomatoes:** Tomatoes are acidic in nature and contain histamines, which can trigger allergic reactions and inflammation in some individuals with eczema.

Tomato-based products like sauces and ketchup may also exacerbate symptoms.

9. **Spices:** Certain spices, such as cinnamon, cloves, and vanilla, can be potential triggers for eczema flare-ups due to their strong flavor compounds and potential allergenic properties.

10. **Artificial Additives:** Artificial additives like preservatives, food dyes, and flavor enhancers found in processed foods, snacks, and beverages can trigger allergic reactions and inflammation in some individuals with eczema.

11. **Alcohol:** Alcohol can dehydrate the body and lead to skin dryness, which may exacerbate eczema symptoms. Additionally, certain types of alcohol, such as red wine and beer, contain histamines and sulfites that can trigger allergic reactions in some individuals.

12. **Processed Foods:** Processed foods high in sugar, refined carbohydrates, trans fats, and artificial additives can exacerbate inflammation in the body and may worsen eczema symptoms. These foods

include fast food, packaged snacks, sugary desserts, and processed meats.

13. **Nightshade Vegetables:** Nightshade vegetables like tomatoes, potatoes, eggplants, and bell peppers contain solanine, a compound that can trigger inflammation and exacerbate eczema symptoms in some individuals.

14. **Caffeine:** Caffeinated beverages like coffee, tea, and energy drinks can dehydrate the body and may exacerbate skin dryness and irritation in individuals with eczema. Additionally, caffeine can stimulate the nervous system and potentially trigger allergic reactions in some people.

TOP ECZEMA SAFE FOODS TO STOP THE ITCH

1. **Fatty Fish:** Fatty fish like salmon, mackerel, and sardines are rich in omega-3 fatty acids, which have anti-inflammatory properties and can help reduce inflammation in the body, including the skin. Incorporating fatty fish into your diet may help alleviate eczema symptoms and reduce itching.

2. **Leafy Greens:** Leafy green vegetables such as spinach, kale, and Swiss chard are packed with vitamins, minerals, and antioxidants that support skin health and reduce inflammation. These nutrient-dense greens can help nourish the skin from within and alleviate eczema symptoms.

3. **Berries:** Berries like strawberries, blueberries, raspberries, and blackberries are rich in antioxidants, particularly vitamin C and flavonoids, which help protect the skin from oxidative stress and inflammation. Including berries in your diet can help support skin health and reduce itching associated with eczema.

4. **Coconut Oil:** Coconut oil is a natural moisturizer with anti-inflammatory and antimicrobial properties that can help soothe and hydrate eczema-prone skin. Consuming coconut oil or using it topically may help alleviate itching and improve skin barrier function in individuals with eczema.

5. **Avocado:** Avocado is rich in healthy fats, vitamins, and antioxidants that support skin health and may help reduce inflammation associated with eczema.

Incorporating avocado into your diet can provide essential nutrients that nourish the skin and alleviate itching.

6. **Probiotic-Rich Foods:** Probiotic-rich foods like yogurt, kefir, sauerkraut, and kimchi contain beneficial bacteria that support gut health and immune function. Maintaining a healthy balance of gut bacteria may help reduce inflammation and improve eczema symptoms, including itching.

7. **Oats:** Oats are a natural skin-soothing ingredient that can help relieve itching and inflammation associated with eczema. Consuming oats in the form of oatmeal or incorporating oat-based products into your diet may help alleviate eczema symptoms and promote skin health.

8. **Turmeric:** Turmeric contains curcumin, a compound with potent anti-inflammatory and antioxidant properties that can help reduce inflammation and itching associated with eczema. Adding turmeric to your diet or consuming it as a supplement may help alleviate eczema symptoms.

9. **Ginger:** Ginger is known for its anti-inflammatory and immune-boosting properties, which can help reduce inflammation and itching in individuals with eczema. Incorporating fresh ginger into your diet or consuming it as a tea may provide relief from eczema symptoms.

10. **Walnuts:** Walnuts are a good source of omega-3 fatty acids and antioxidants, which can help reduce inflammation and support skin health. Including walnuts in your diet may help alleviate itching and improve eczema symptoms.

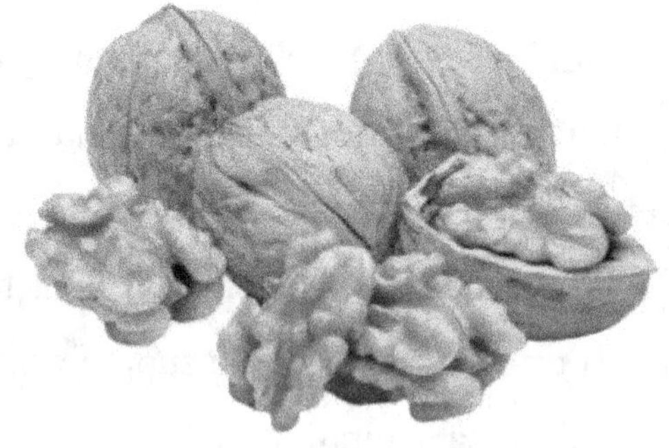

CHAPTER 2

14-DAY MEAL PLAN

DAY 1

Breakfast: Quinoa Porridge with Berries

Lunch: Quinoa Salad with Avocado

Dinner: Grilled Chicken with Quinoa Pilaf

DAY 2

Breakfast: Gluten-Free Oatmeal with Chia Seeds and Turmeric

Lunch: Lentil Bowl with Spinach and Carrots

Dinner: Baked Salmon with Roasted Vegetables

DAY 3

Breakfast: Brown Rice Breakfast Bowl with Spinach and Avocado

Lunch: Zucchini Noodles with Pesto

Dinner: Roasted Chicken with Sweet Potato and Broccoli

DAY 4

Breakfast: Unsalted Rice Cake with Smashed Avocado

Lunch: Turkey Lettuce Wraps with Cucumber and Carrot Slaw

Dinner: Zucchini Noodles with Pesto

DAY 5

Breakfast: Coconut Flour Pancakes with Blueberry Compote

Lunch: Baked Chicken with Roasted Sweet Potatoes and Green Beans

Dinner: Grilled Shrimp and Vegetable Skewers

DAY 6

Breakfast: Polenta Porridge with Apples

Lunch: Grilled Vegetable Quinoa Bowl with Tahini Dressing

Dinner: Baked Cod with Herbs

DAY 7

Breakfast: Teff Porridge with Mango and Coconut

Lunch: Eggplant and Bell Pepper Casserole with Herbs

Dinner: Baked Chicken with Roasted Brussels Sprouts

DAY 8

Breakfast: Oat Flour Frittata with Spinach and Bell Pepper

Lunch: Spinach and Mushroom Quiche with Gluten-Free Crust

Dinner: Stir-Fried Quinoa with Mixed Vegetables

DAY 9

Breakfast: Buckwheat Banana Bread

Lunch: Turkey and Vegetable Soup with Quinoa

Dinner: Baked Turkey Meatballs with Zucchini Noodles

DAY 10

Breakfast: Rice Flake Porridge with Caramelized Banana

Lunch: Chickpea Salad with Cucumber and Bell Pepper

Dinner: Grilled Shrimp and Vegetable Skewers

DAY 11

Breakfast: Quinoa Porridge with Berries

Lunch: Quinoa Salad with Avocado

Dinner: Grilled Chicken with Quinoa Pilaf

DAY 12

Breakfast: Gluten-Free Oatmeal with Chia Seeds and Turmeric

Lunch: Lentil Bowl with Spinach and Carrots

Dinner: Baked Salmon with Roasted Vegetables

DAY 13

Breakfast: Brown Rice Breakfast Bowl with Spinach and Avocado

Lunch: Zucchini Noodles with Pesto

Dinner: Roasted Chicken with Sweet Potato and Broccoli

DAY 14

Breakfast: Unsalted Rice Cake with Smashed Avocado

Lunch: Turkey Lettuce Wraps with Cucumber and Carrot Slaw

Dinner: Zucchini Noodles with Pesto

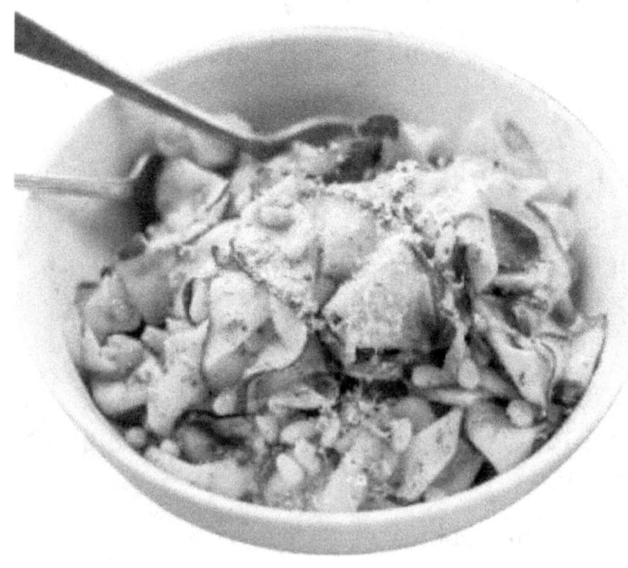

CHAPTER 3

NUTRITIOUS RECIPES FOR AN ECZEMA DIET

BREAKFAST

Quinoa Porridge with Berries

Preparation Time: 25 minutes

Serves: 2

Calories: 350 **Sodium:** 50mg **Sugar:** 4g

Ingredients:

1 cup quinoa

2 cups water

1 cup coconut milk (or any non-dairy milk)

1 tablespoon honey (or maple syrup)

1 cup mixed berries (such as strawberries, blueberries, raspberries)

2 tablespoons pumpkin seeds (or sunflower seeds), for garnish

Method of Method of Preparation:

1. Rinse the quinoa under cold water.
2. In a medium saucepan, combine quinoa and water.
3. Bring to a boil, then reduce heat to low and simmer for 15-20 minutes, until quinoa is cooked and water is absorbed.
4. Stir in coconut milk, and honey.
5. Cook for another 5 minutes, stirring occasionally.
6. Serve hot, topped with mixed berries and pumpkin seeds.

Gluten-Free Oatmeal with Chia Seeds and Turmeric

Preparation Time: 15 minutes

Serves: 2

Calories: 300 **Sodium:** 5mg **Sugar:** 4g

Ingredients:

1 cup gluten-free rolled oats

2 cups water

1 tablespoon chia seeds

1 teaspoon ground turmeric

1 tablespoon honey (or maple syrup)

1/2 cup sliced banana

2 tablespoons shredded coconut, for garnish

Method of Method of Preparation:

1. In a saucepan, bring water to a boil.
2. Add oats, chia seeds, and turmeric.
3. Reduce heat to low and simmer for 5-7 minutes, stirring occasionally.
4. Stir in honey and sliced banana.
5. Cook for another 2-3 minutes until the oatmeal reaches your desired consistency.
6. Serve hot, garnished with shredded coconut.

Brown Rice Breakfast Bowl with Spinach and Avocado

Preparation Time: 20 minutes

Serves: 2

Calories: 350 **Sodium:** 150mg **Sugar:** 1g

Ingredients:

1 cup cooked brown rice

1 cup fresh spinach leaves

1/2 avocado, sliced

1 tablespoon olive oil

Pepper

Method of Method of Preparation:

1. In a bowl, layer cooked brown rice, fresh spinach leaves, and sliced avocado.
2. Drizzle with olive oil and season with pepper.
3. Serve immediately.

Unsalted Rice Cake with Smashed Avocado

Preparation Time: 10 minutes

Serves: 2

Calories: 200 **Sodium:** 10mg **Sugar:** 1g

Ingredients:

2 rice cakes

1 avocado, mashed

1 tablespoon lemon juice

1 tablespoon hemp seeds, for garnish

Fresh basil leaves, for garnish

Method of Method of Preparation:

1. Spread mashed avocado evenly on each rice cake.
2. Drizzle with lemon juice.
3. Garnish with hemp seeds and fresh basil leaves.
4. Serve immediately.

Coconut Flour Pancakes with Blueberry Compote

Preparation Time: 20 minutes

Serves: 4

Calories: 250 **Sodium:** 100mg **Sugar:** 8g

Ingredients:

1/2 cup coconut flour

1 cup coconut milk

1 tablespoon honey (or maple syrup)

1 teaspoon vanilla extract

1/2 teaspoon baking powder (gluten-free)

1 cup fresh blueberries

1 tablespoon lemon juice

1 tablespoon water

Method of Method of Preparation:

1. In a mixing bowl, whisk together coconut flour, coconut milk, honey, vanilla extract, and baking powder until smooth.
2. Heat a non-stick skillet over medium heat.
3. Pour 1/4 cup of batter onto the skillet for each pancake.
4. Cook until bubbles form on the surface, then flip and cook until golden brown on the other side.

5. In a saucepan, combine blueberries, lemon juice, and water.

6. Cook over medium heat until the blueberries break down and form a compote.

7. Serve pancakes topped with blueberry compote.

Polenta Porridge with Apples

Preparation Time: 25 minutes

Serves: 2

Calories: 300 **Sodium:** 5mg **Sugar:** 10g

Ingredients:

1 cup polenta

3 cups water

2 apples, diced

1 tablespoon honey (optional, for sweetness)

Method of Preparation:

1. In a saucepan, bring the water to a boil.

2. Slowly whisk in the polenta and reduce the heat to low.

3. Simmer, stirring occasionally, for 15-20 minutes until the polenta is thick and creamy.

4. In a separate pan, sauté the diced apples until they are soft and caramelized.

5. Serve the polenta porridge topped with the caramelized apples.

6. Drizzle with honey if desired.

Teff Porridge with Mango and Coconut

Preparation Time: 25 minutes

Serves: 2

Calories: 350 **Sodium:** 2mg **Sugar:** 15g

Ingredients:

1 cup teff grains

2 cups water

1 ripe mango, diced

2 tablespoons shredded coconut

Method of Preparation:

1. Rinse the teff grains under cold water.
2. In a saucepan, bring the water to a boil, then add the teff grains.
3. Reduce the heat to low and simmer for 15-20 minutes, stirring occasionally, until the teff is tender and the water is absorbed.
4. Serve the teff porridge topped with diced mango and shredded coconut.

Oat Flour Frittata with Spinach and Bell Peppers

Preparation Time: 35 minutes

Serves: 4

Calories: 180 **Sodium:** 100mg **Sugar:** 2g

Ingredients:

1 cup oat flour

1 1/2 cups water

1 cup chopped spinach

1/2 cup diced bell peppers

1 teaspoon turmeric powder

Method of Preparation:

1. Preheat the oven to 375°F (190°C).
2. In a bowl, whisk together the oat flour, water, turmeric powder, until smooth.
3. Stir in the chopped spinach and diced bell peppers.
4. Pour the mixture into a greased baking dish.
5. Bake for 25-30 minutes until the frittata is set and golden brown on top.
6. Slice and serve warm.

Buckwheat Banana Bread

Preparation Time: 50 minutes

Serves: 8

Calories: 200 **Sodium:** 50mg **Sugar:** 8g

Ingredients:

2 ripe bananas, mashed

1 cup buckwheat flour

1/4 cup honey

1/4 cup coconut oil, melted

1 teaspoon baking powder

Method of Preparation:

1. Preheat the oven to 350°F (175°C).
2. In a large bowl, combine the mashed bananas, honey, melted coconut oil, and eggs.
3. Stir in the buckwheat flour, and baking powder until well combined.
4. Pour the batter into a greased loaf pan.
5. Bake for 40-45 minutes until a toothpick inserted into the center comes out clean.
6. Allow the banana bread to cool before slicing and serving.

Rice Flake Porridge with Caramelized Banana

Preparation Time: 15 minutes

Serves: 2

Calories: 250 **Sodium:** 10mg **Sugar:** 12g

Ingredients:

1 cup rice flakes

2 cups coconut milk

2 ripe bananas, sliced

2 tablespoons coconut sugar

Method of Preparation:

1. In a saucepan, bring the coconut milk to a simmer.
2. Stir in the rice flakes and cook for 5-7 minutes until the porridge thickens.
3. In a separate pan, heat the coconut sugar over medium heat until it melts and caramelizes.
4. Add the sliced bananas to the caramelized sugar and cook until they are golden brown.
5. Serve the rice flake porridge topped with the caramelized bananas.

LUNCH

Quinoa Salad with Avocado

Preparation Time: 20 minutes

Serves: 4

Calories: 290 **Sodium:** 10mg **Sugar:** 2g

Ingredients:

1 cup quinoa, rinsed

2 cups water

1 avocado, diced

1/4 cup fresh cilantro, chopped

2 tablespoons extra virgin olive oil

Black pepper

Method of Preparation:

1. In a medium saucepan, combine quinoa and water.
2. Bring to a boil, then reduce heat to low, cover, and simmer for 15 minutes, or until quinoa is cooked and water is absorbed.
3. Remove from heat and let it cool.
4. In a large bowl, combine cooked quinoa, diced avocado and chopped cilantro.
5. In a small bowl, whisk together olive oil. Pour over the quinoa salad and toss gently to combine.

6. Season with salt and black pepper to taste.

7. Serve chilled or at room temperature.

Lentil Bowl with Spinach and Carrots

Preparation Time: 30 minutes

Serves: 4

Calories: 230 **Sodium:** 200mg **Sugar:** 3g

Ingredients:

1 cup green lentils, rinsed

2 cups vegetable broth

2 cups spinach leaves

1 cup carrots, grated

1 tablespoon extra-virgin olive oil

2 cloves garlic, minced

1 teaspoon ground cumin

1/2 teaspoon ground turmeric

Black pepper to taste

Method of Preparation:

1. In a medium saucepan, combine lentils and vegetable broth.
2. Bring to a boil, then reduce heat to low, cover, and simmer for 20-25 minutes, or until lentils are tender.
3. In a large skillet, heat olive oil over medium heat.
4. Add minced garlic and cook for 1-2 minutes, until fragrant.
5. Add grated carrots to the skillet and cook for 3-4 minutes, until softened.
6. Stir in spinach leaves and cook until wilted.
7. Add cooked lentils to the skillet and sprinkle with ground cumin and turmeric.
8. Stir to combine and heat through.
9. Season with black pepper.
10. Serve hot.

Zucchini Noodles with Pesto

Preparation Time: 15 minutes

Serves: 4

Calories: 150 **Sodium:** 120mg **Sugar:** 4g

Ingredients:

4 medium zucchinis, spiralized into noodles

1/4 cup basil pesto (made with olive oil, basil, garlic, and nutritional yeast instead of cheese)

2 tablespoons pine nuts (optional, omit if nut-free)

Black pepper to taste

Method of Preparation:

1. In a large skillet, heat a drizzle of olive oil over medium heat.
2. Add zucchini noodles.
3. Cook for 3-4 minutes, until zucchini noodles are tender.
4. Stir in basil pesto and pine nuts (if using).
5. Cook for an additional 1-2 minutes, until heated through.
6. Season with black pepper.
7. Serve hot.

Turkey Lettuce Wraps with Cucumber and Carrot Slaw

Preparation Time: 35 minutes

Serves: 4

Calories: 320 **Sodium:** 90mg **Sugar:** 5g

Preparation Time: 25 minutes

Serves: 4

Calories: 270 **Sodium:** 70mg **Sugar:** 3g

Ingredients:

1 lb. ground turkey

1 tablespoon olive oil

1 teaspoon ground cumin

1 teaspoon paprika

1 teaspoon garlic powder

1 cup cucumber, julienned

1 cup carrots, julienned

1/4 cup fresh cilantro, chopped

Juice of 1 lime

Black pepper to taste

Butter lettuce leaves, for serving

Method of Preparation:

1. In a large skillet, heat olive oil over medium heat.
2. Add ground turkey and cook until browned, breaking it apart with a spatula.
3. Stir in ground cumin, paprika, and garlic powder.
4. Cook for an additional 2-3 minutes, until fragrant.
5. In a medium bowl, combine julienned cucumber, carrots, chopped cilantro, and lime juice.
6. Toss to combine.
7. Season turkey mixture with black pepper.
8. To assemble, spoon turkey mixture onto butter lettuce leaves and top with cucumber and carrot slaw.
9. Serve immediately.

Baked Chicken with Roasted Sweet Potatoes and Green Beans

Ingredients:

4 boneless, skinless chicken breasts

2 sweet potatoes, peeled and cubed

2 cups green beans, trimmed

2 tablespoons olive oil

1 teaspoon dried thyme

1 teaspoon garlic powder

Black pepper to taste

Method of Preparation:

1. Preheat oven to 400°F (200°C).
2. Place chicken breasts on a baking sheet lined with parchment paper.
3. Drizzle with olive oil and sprinkle with dried thyme, garlic powder, salt, and black pepper.
4. Arrange cubed sweet potatoes and green beans around the chicken on the baking sheet.

5. Drizzle with olive oil and season with black pepper.

6. Bake in the preheated oven for 20-25 minutes, or until chicken is cooked through and vegetables are tender.

7. Serve hot.

Grilled Vegetable Quinoa Bowl with Tahini Dressing

Preparation Time: 30 minutes

Serves: 4

Calories: 320 **Sodium:** 20mg **Sugar:** 4g

Ingredients:

1 cup quinoa

2 cups water

1 medium eggplant, sliced

1 medium zucchini, sliced

1 red bell pepper, sliced

1 yellow bell pepper, sliced

1 tablespoon olive oil

¼ cup tahini

Water (as needed to thin dressing)

Fresh parsley for garnish

Method of Preparation:

1. Rinse quinoa under cold water.
2. In a medium saucepan, combine quinoa and water.
3. Bring to a boil, then reduce heat to low, cover, and simmer for 15-20 minutes until water is absorbed and quinoa is tender.
4. Remove from heat and let it sit covered for 5 minutes.
5. Fluff with a fork.
6. Preheat grill to medium-high heat.
7. Brush eggplant, zucchini, and bell peppers with olive oil.
8. Grill vegetables until tender and lightly charred, about 5-7 minutes per side.
9. In a small bowl, whisk together tahini and water until smooth.

10. Add more water as needed to achieve desired consistency for the dressing.

11. To assemble bowls, divide cooked quinoa among serving bowls.

12. Top with grilled vegetables and drizzle with tahini dressing.

13. Garnish with fresh parsley.

Eggplant and Bell Pepper Casserole with Herbs

Preparation Time: 45 minutes

Serves: 4

Calories: 120 **Sodium:** 10mg **Sugar:** 6g

Ingredients:

2 medium eggplants, sliced

2 large bell peppers, sliced

2 tablespoons olive oil

1 teaspoon dried thyme

1 teaspoon dried oregano

Fresh basil leaves for garnish

Method of Preparation:

1. Preheat oven to 375°F (190°C).

2. Grease a baking dish with olive oil.

3. Arrange eggplant and bell pepper slices in the baking dish, alternating layers.

4. Sprinkle dried thyme, and dried oregano evenly over the layers.

5. Drizzle with olive oil.

6. Cover the dish with foil and bake for 30 minutes.

7. Remove foil and bake for an additional 15-20 minutes until vegetables are tender and lightly browned.

8. Garnish with fresh basil leaves before serving.

Spinach and Mushroom Quiche with Gluten-Free Crust

Preparation Time: 1 hour

Serves: 6

Calories: 180 **Sodium:** 150mg **Sugar:** 2g

Ingredients:

1 gluten-free pie crust (store-bought or homemade)

2 cups fresh spinach, chopped

1 cup mushrooms, sliced

1 small onion, diced

1 cup coconut milk (or any non-dairy milk)

Fresh parsley for garnish

Method of Preparation:

1. Preheat oven to 375°F (190°C).
2. Place gluten-free pie crust in a pie dish and set aside.
3. In a skillet, sauté chopped spinach, mushrooms, and diced onion until vegetables are tender and any excess moisture has evaporated.
4. Season with pepper.
5. Add coconut milk, make sure it is thick enough.
6. Spread sautéed vegetables evenly over the bottom of the pie crust.
7. Pour coconut milk over the vegetables.

8.   Bake quiche for 30-35 minutes until set and golden brown on top.

9.   Allow to cool slightly before slicing.

10. Garnish with fresh parsley.

Turkey and Vegetable Soup with Quinoa

Preparation Time: 40 minutes

Serves: 6

Calories: 280 **Sodium:** 200mg **Sugar:** 4g

Ingredients:

1 tablespoon olive oil

1 onion, diced

2 carrots, diced

2 stalks celery, diced

1 lb. ground turkey

6 cups low-sodium chicken broth

1 cup quinoa

2 bay leaves

Fresh parsley for garnish

Method of Preparation:

1. In a large pot, heat olive oil over medium heat.
2. Add diced onion, carrots, celery, and minced garlic.
3. Sauté until vegetables are tender.
4. Add ground turkey to the pot and cook until browned, breaking it apart with a spoon.
5. Pour in chicken broth and add quinoa and bay leaves.
6. Bring to a boil, then reduce heat and simmer for 20-25 minutes until quinoa is cooked and vegetables are tender.
7. Season with pepper if desired.
8. Remove bay leaves before serving.
9. Garnish with fresh parsley.

Chickpea Salad with Cucumber and Bell Pepper

Preparation Time: 15 minutes

Serves: 4

Calories: 260 **Sodium:** 150mg **Sugar:** 6g

Ingredients:

2 cans (15 oz each) chickpeas, rinsed and drained

1 cucumber, diced

2 bell pepper, diced

¼ cup fresh parsley, chopped

¼ cup olive oil

1 teaspoon ground cumin

Salt and pepper to taste (optional, can be omitted)

Method of Preparation:

1. In a large bowl, combine chickpeas, diced cucumber, diced bell pepper, and chopped parsley.
2. In a small bowl, whisk together olive oil, lemon juice, and ground cumin to make the dressing.
3. Pour the dressing over the chickpea mixture and toss until well coated.
4. Season with salt and pepper if desired.
5. Serve chilled or at room temperature.

DINNER

Grilled Chicken with Quinoa Pilaf

Preparation Time: 25 minutes

Serves: 4

Calories: 350 **Sodium:** 250mg **Sugar:** 3g

Ingredients:

4 boneless, skinless chicken breasts

2 tablespoons olive oil

1 teaspoon dried oregano

1 teaspoon dried thyme

1 cup quinoa, rinsed and drained

2 cups low-sodium vegetable broth

1 cup chopped fresh spinach

Method of Preparation:

1. Preheat grill to medium-high heat.
2. In a small bowl, whisk together olive oil, oregano, and thyme.

3. Brush chicken breasts with the mixture and let marinate for 10 minutes.

4. Grill chicken breasts for 6-8 minutes per side or until cooked through.

5. In a medium saucepan, bring vegetable broth to a boil.

6. Stir in quinoa, reduce heat to low, cover, and simmer for 15-20 minutes or until quinoa is cooked and liquid is absorbed.

7. Fluff cooked quinoa with a fork and stir in chopped spinach.

8. Serve grilled chicken alongside quinoa pilaf.

Baked Salmon with Roasted Vegetables

Preparation Time: 35 minutes

Serves: 4

Calories: 320 **Sodium:** 180mg **Sugar:** 6g

Ingredients:

4 salmon fillets

2 tablespoons olive oil

1 teaspoon dried dill

1 teaspoon dried parsley

1 teaspoon garlic powder

2 cups mixed vegetables, chopped

Method of Preparation:

1. Preheat oven to 400°F (200°C).
2. Place salmon fillets on a baking sheet lined with parchment paper.
3. In a small bowl, mix together olive oil, dill and parsley.
4. Brush mixture over salmon fillets.
5. Arrange mixed vegetables around salmon on the baking sheet.
6. Bake for 15-20 minutes or until salmon is cooked through and vegetables are tender.
7. Serve baked salmon with roasted vegetables.

Roasted Chicken with Sweet Potato and Broccoli

Preparation Time: 20 minutes

Serves: 4

Calories: 250 **Sodium:** 150mg **Sugar:** 4g

Ingredients:

4 chicken thighs, bone-in and skin-on

2 tablespoons olive oil

1 teaspoon paprika

1 teaspoon dried rosemary

2 sweet potatoes, peeled and diced

2 cups broccoli florets

Method of Preparation:

1. Preheat oven to 400°F (200°C).
2. Place chicken thighs on a baking sheet lined with parchment paper.

3. In a small bowl, mix together olive oil, paprika, and dried rosemary.

4. Brush mixture over chicken thighs.

5. Arrange diced sweet potatoes and broccoli florets around chicken on the baking sheet.

6. Bake for 25-30 minutes or until chicken is cooked through and vegetables are tender.

7. Serve roasted chicken with sweet potatoes and broccoli.

Zucchini Noodles with Pesto

Preparation Time: 20 minutes

Serves: 4

Calories: 180 **Sodium:** 220mg **Sugar:** 3g

Ingredients:

4 medium zucchinis, spiralized into noodles

Bell peppers

1/4 cup pesto sauce

Method of Preparation:

1. In a large skillet, heat olive oil over medium heat.

2. Add zucchini noodles and bell pepper to the skillet.

3. Cook for 3-4 minutes or until vegetables are tender.

4. Stir in pesto sauce and cook for an additional 1-2 minutes.

5. Serve immediately.

Grilled Shrimp and Vegetable Skewers

Preparation Time: 30 minutes

Serves: 3

Calories: 100 **Sodium:** 90mg **Sugar:** 0g

Ingredients:

16 large shrimp, peeled and deveined

2 bell peppers, cut into chunks

1 red onion, cut into chunks

1 zucchini, sliced

2 tablespoons olive oil

1 teaspoon smoked paprika

1 teaspoon dried thyme

Method of Preparation:

1. Preheat grill to medium-high heat.
2. Thread shrimp, bell peppers, red onion, and zucchini onto skewers.
3. In a small bowl, mix together olive oil, smoked paprika, and dried thyme.
4. Brush mixture over skewers.
5. Grill skewers for 3-4 minutes per side or until shrimp is pink and vegetables are tender.
6. Serve grilled shrimp and vegetable skewers.

Baked Cod with Herbs

Preparation time: 25 minutes

Serves: 4

Calories: 220 **Sodium:** 75mg **Sugar:** 0g

Ingredients:

4 cod fillets

2 tablespoons olive oil

2 tablespoons fresh parsley, chopped

1 teaspoon dried thyme

Method of Preparation:

1. Preheat the oven to 400°F (200°C).
2. Place the cod fillets in a baking dish.
3. Drizzle the olive oil over the cod fillets.
4. Sprinkle chopped parsley, dried thyme, and pepper evenly over the fillets.
5. Bake in the preheated oven for 15-20 minutes, or until the fish is cooked through and flakes easily with a fork.
6. Serve hot.

Baked Chicken with Roasted Brussels Sprouts

Preparation time: 35 minutes

Serves: 4

Calories: 320 **Sodium:** 95mg **Sugar:** 2g

Ingredients:

4 chicken breasts

2 tablespoons olive oil

1 teaspoon paprika

1 teaspoon dried thyme

1 pound Brussels sprouts, halved

Method of Preparation:

1. Preheat the oven to 400°F (200°C).
2. Place the chicken breasts in a baking dish.
3. Drizzle olive oil over the chicken breasts.
4. Sprinkle paprika, dried thyme, and pepper evenly over the chicken breasts.
5. Arrange the Brussels sprouts around the chicken in the baking dish.
6. Bake in the preheated oven for 25-30 minutes, or until the chicken is cooked through and the Brussels sprouts are tender.
7. Serve hot.

Stir-Fried Quinoa with Mixed Vegetables

Preparation time: 30 minutes

Serves: 4

Calories: 220 **Sodium:** 410mg **Sugar:** 6g

Ingredients:

Quinoa

2 tablespoons olive oil

1 cup broccoli florets

1 bell pepper, sliced

1 carrot, sliced

2 tablespoons soy sauce (or tamari for gluten-free)

1 teaspoon sesame oil

Method of Preparation:

1. Heat olive oil in a large skillet over medium heat.
2. Add quinoa and stir-fry.
3. Add broccoli, bell pepper, carrot, and to the skillet.

4. Stir-fry until vegetables are tender-crisp.

5. Add sesame oil, toss to combine.

6. Cook for another 2-3 minutes.

7. Serve hot.

Baked Turkey Meatballs with Zucchini Noodles

Preparation time: 40 minutes

Serves: 4

Calories: 280 **Sodium:** 480mg **Sugar:** 6g

Ingredients:

1 pound ground turkey

1/2 cup gluten-free breadcrumbs

2 cloves garlic, minced

1 teaspoon dried oregano

1/2 teaspoon dried basil

Bell pepper

2 large zucchinis, spiralized into noodles

Method of Preparation:

1. Preheat the oven to 400°F (200°C).

2. In a large bowl, combine ground turkey, gluten-free breadcrumbs dried oregano, dried basil, and pepper.

3. Mix until well combined, then form the mixture into meatballs.

4. Place the meatballs on a baking sheet lined with parchment paper.

5. Bake in the preheated oven for 20-25 minutes, or until cooked through.

6. While the meatballs are baking, heat the bell pepper sauce in a skillet over medium heat.

7. Add the zucchini noodles to the skillet and toss until heated through.

8. Serve the baked turkey meatballs on top of the zucchini noodles with bell pepper sauce.

DESSERTS

Baked Apples

Preparation Time: 40 minutes

Serves: 4

Calories: 120 **Sodium:** 0mg **Sugar:** 20g

Ingredients:

4 large apples, cored

1 tablespoon honey (or maple syrup for vegan option)

Method of Preparation:

1. Preheat the oven to 375°F (190°C).
2. Place the cored apples in a baking dish.
3. Sprinkle each apple with honey.
4. Bake for 30 minutes, or until the apples are tender.
5. Serve warm.

Mango Sorbet

Preparation Time: 5 minutes + Freezing Time: 4 hours

Serves: 4

Calories: 120 **Sodium:** 0mg **Sugar:** 28g

Ingredients:

4 ripe mangoes, peeled and diced

2 tablespoons honey (or maple syrup for vegan option)

Method of Preparation:

1. Place the diced mangoes in a blender or food processor.
2. Add honey.
3. Blend until smooth.
4. Pour the mixture into a shallow dish and freeze for at least 4 hours, or until firm.
5. Serve chilled.

Avocado Chocolate Mousse

Preparation Time: 10 minutes

Serves: 4

Calories: 220 **Sodium:** 10mg **Sugar:** 14g

Ingredients:

2 ripe avocados, peeled and pitted

1/4 cup cocoa powder

1/4 cup honey (or maple syrup for vegan option)

1 teaspoon vanilla extract

Method of Preparation:

1. Place the avocados, cocoa powder, honey, and vanilla extract in a blender or food processor.
2. Blend until smooth and creamy.
3. Chill in the refrigerator for at least 30 minutes before serving.
4. Serve chilled.

Steamed Pears with Honey and Cinnamon

Preparation Time: 30 minutes

Serves: 4

Calories: 100 **Sodium:** 0mg **Sugar:** 20g

Ingredients:

4 ripe pears, peeled and cored

2 tablespoons honey (or maple syrup for vegan option)

Method of Preparation:

1. Place a steamer basket in a pot filled with water.
2. Bring the water to a boil over medium heat.

3. Place the pears in the steamer basket, cover, and steam for 15 minutes, or until tender.

4. Remove the pears from the steamer basket and place them on serving plates.

5. Drizzle with honey.

6. Serve warm.

Carrot Cake Bites

Preparation Time: 15 minutes

Serves: 12

Calories: 120 **Sodium:** 5mg **Sugar:** 10g

Ingredients:

2 cups grated carrots

1 cup rolled oats

1/2 cup dates, pitted

1/4 cup shredded coconut

1/2 teaspoon ground ginger

1 tablespoon honey (or maple syrup for vegan option)

Method of Preparation:

1. Place all ingredients in a food processor.
2. Pulse until well combined and the mixture sticks together.
3. Roll the mixture into small balls.
4. Place the balls on a baking sheet lined with parchment paper.
5. Chill in the refrigerator for at least 30 minutes before serving.
6. Serve chilled.

SOUPS AND STEWS

Turmeric Carrot Soup

Preparation Time: 30 minutes

Serves: 6

Calories: 120 **Sodium:** 600mg **Sugar:** 10g

Ingredients:

1 tablespoon olive oil

1 onion, chopped

1 tablespoon grated fresh ginger

1 teaspoon ground turmeric

1 teaspoon ground cumin

1/2 teaspoon ground coriander

1/4 teaspoon cayenne pepper (optional)

1 kg carrots, peeled and chopped

4 cups vegetable broth

Freshly ground black pepper, to taste

Fresh cilantro, for garnish

Method of Preparation:

1. In a large pot, heat olive oil over medium heat.
2. Add the onion and cook until translucent, about 5 minutes.
3. Add the ginger, turmeric, cumin, coriander, and cayenne pepper (if using).
4. Cook for another 2 minutes, stirring constantly.
5. Add the chopped carrots and vegetable broth.
6. Bring to a boil, then reduce heat and simmer until the carrots are tender, about 20 minutes.

7. Use an immersion blender to puree the soup until smooth.

8. Season with black pepper.

9. Serve hot, garnished with fresh cilantro.

Butternut Squash Soup

Preparation Time: 40 minutes

Serves: 6

Calories: 150 **Sodium:** 500mg **Sugar:** 8g

Ingredients:

1 tablespoon olive oil

1 onion, chopped

1 butternut squash, peeled, seeded, and chopped

4 cups vegetable broth

Freshly ground black pepper, to taste

Fresh parsley, for garnish

Method of Preparation:

1. In a large pot, heat olive oil over medium heat.

2. Add the onion and cook until translucent, about 5 minutes.

3. Add the chopped butternut squash and vegetable broth.

4. Bring to a boil, then reduce heat and simmer until the squash is tender, about 20 minutes.

5. Use an immersion blender to puree the soup until smooth.

6. Season with black pepper.

7. Serve hot, garnished with fresh parsley.

Chicken and Vegetable Soup

Preparation Time: 40 minutes

Serves: 6

Calories: 200 **Sodium:** 700mg **Sugar:** 4g

Ingredients:

1 tablespoon olive oil

1 onion, chopped

2 carrots, peeled and chopped

2 celery stalks, chopped

1 zucchini, chopped

1 kg boneless, skinless chicken breasts, cut into bite-sized pieces

6 cups chicken broth

1 teaspoon dried thyme

1 teaspoon dried oregano

Freshly ground black pepper, to taste

Fresh parsley, for garnish

Method of Preparation:

1. In a large pot, heat olive oil over medium heat.
2. Add the onion and cook until translucent, about 5 minutes.
3. Add the garlic and cook for another 2 minutes, stirring constantly.
4. Add the carrots, celery, zucchini, chicken, chicken broth, thyme, and oregano.
5. Bring to a boil, then reduce heat and simmer until the chicken is cooked through and the vegetables are tender, about 20 minutes.

6. Season with black pepper.

7. Serve hot, garnished with fresh parsley.

Lentil Soup with Spinach

Ingredients:

1 tablespoon olive oil

1 onion, chopped

2 carrots, peeled and chopped

2 celery stalks, chopped

1 cup dried green lentils, rinsed

6 cups vegetable broth

2 cups fresh spinach

1 teaspoon dried thyme

1 teaspoon dried rosemary

Freshly ground black pepper

Method of Preparation:

1. In a large pot, heat olive oil over medium heat.

2. Add the onion and cook until translucent, about 5 minutes.

3. Add the garlic and cook for another 2 minutes, stirring constantly.

4. Add the carrots, celery, lentils, vegetable broth, thyme, and rosemary.

5. Bring to a boil, then reduce heat and simmer until the lentils are tender, about 30 minutes.

6. Stir in the spinach and cook until wilted, about 5 minutes.

7. Season with black pepper.

8. Serve hot.

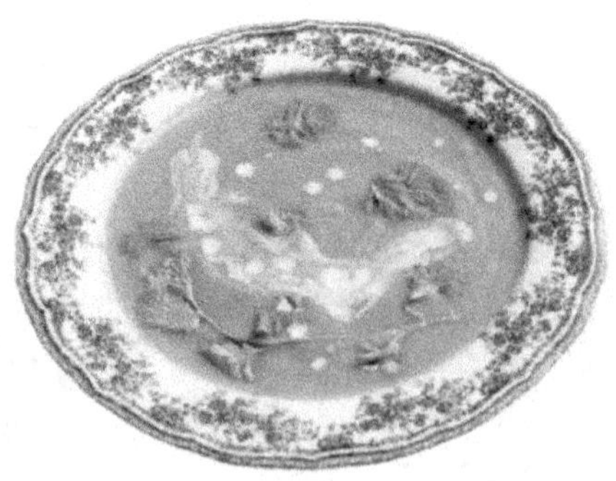

CONCLUSION

In conclusion, this cookbook offers a comprehensive guide to managing eczema symptoms through mindful dietary choices and nourishing recipes.

Throughout the pages of this book, you've explored the intricate relationship between food and eczema, uncovering the power of anti-inflammatory ingredients and eczema-safe foods to alleviate itching, reduce inflammation, and promote overall skin health.

By embracing the principles of the eczema diet, you have embarked on a journey of healing and self-discovery, learning to identify trigger foods, optimize gut health, and nourish our body with nutrient-rich, skin-nourishing ingredients.

Beyond the kitchen, this cookbook serves as a valuable resource for understanding the underlying mechanisms of eczema and the role that diet plays in its management.

With each delicious chew, may you find relief from itching, comfort in nourishment, and joy in the simple act of nourishing your body with wholesome, eczema-safe ingredients.

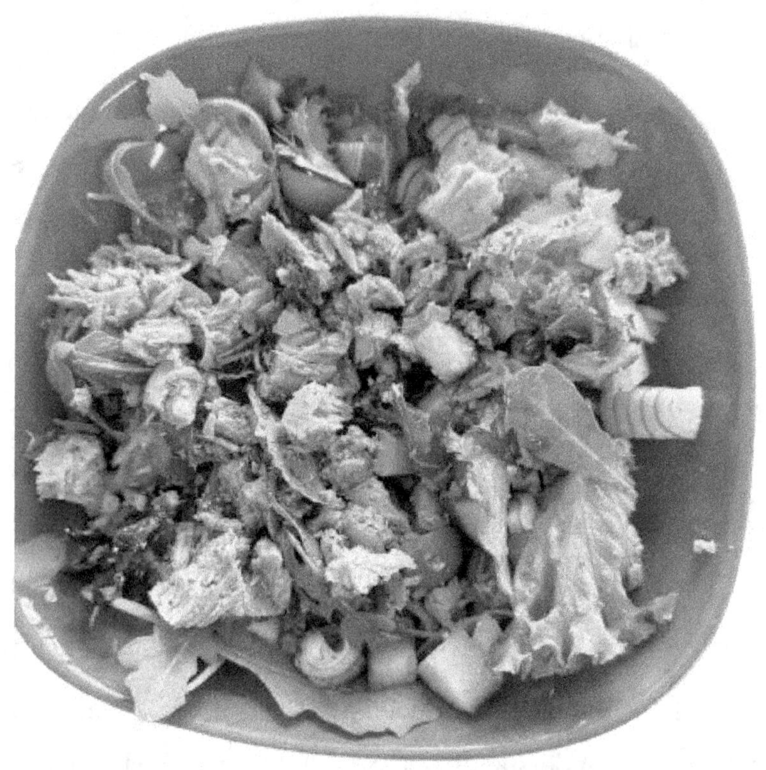